TEN CARDINAL SECRETS FOR LOSING WEIGHT AFTER 40 YEARS

A Concise Guide for Women to Achieve Hormone Balance and Lose Weight after 40 Years

James Edwards

TABLE OF CONTENTS

INTRODUCTION

This book is a concise guide that will give you the wisdom you need to handle the frequently confusing and complicated world of weight control, especially after the age of forty years.

The turning of forty is a big deal for a lot of individuals. It brings with it new difficulties and adjustments, particularly in terms of keeping a healthy weight. Hormones change, the metabolism slows down, and lifestyle variables may become more ingrained. Amidst all these hindrances, it may seem impractical to sustain your fitness and achieve the goal of losing weight.

But this book isn't about short cures or implausible novelty diets. Rather, it dives deeply into the essential ideas and techniques that will enable you to effectively and soundly take charge of your weight and well-being.

We'll look at the particular difficulties that people over forty have when trying to lose weight in the opening section. Developing a successful weight loss plan requires a comprehension of these variables, which range from metabolic alterations to muscle loss and elevated stress levels.

The book's ensuing section is devoted to hormones and how they affect weight gain and loss. Hormones are important participants in the weight control strategy since they control hunger, energy levels, and metabolism. Gaining knowledge of the roles of hormones in weight loss and how lifestyle decisions affect them can provide you with the wisdom you need to maximize your weight loss endeavors.

You'll find useful revelations, evidence-based tactics, and realistic recommendations all over this book that you may incorporate into your everyday routine. To assist in your weight loss objectives, every facet of holistic health and fitness is covered, from exercise and diet to stress control and sleep enhancement.

'Ten Cardinal Secrets for Losing Weight After 40' is your reliable guide to more satisfying body weight, regardless of whether you're starting your weight loss venture from scratch or want to pick up where you left off. Together, let's set out on this life-changing adventure to discover the keys to long-term weight loss and robust health beyond forty years of age.

CHAPTER ONE

The Secret of Mindful Eating

In the pursuit of reducing weight after the age of forty, mindful eating is a potent mechanism that can make a big difference in our progress. Eating mindfully involves not solely the things we consume but also how we consume them. It's about learning to recognize our bodies' signals of hunger and fullness, comprehending the emotions that are associated with eating, and forming a more positive connection with the food we eat.

The exercise of mindful eating has its roots in mindfulness, which is the deliberate, judgment-free attention to the here and now. This follows that when we relate it to eating, we have to be completely conscious of what we are eating, how it makes us feel, and how it affects our body and mood.

This strategy invites us to take our time, enjoy every bite, and concentrate on our bodies' signals of starvation and fullness. By doing this, we can overcome mindless eating behaviors including eating rapidly, eating when upset, or eating during the time that you're preoccupied.

Five Advantages of Mindful Eating

1. Increased Awareness: Mindful eating makes us more conscious of our eating patterns, particularly restlessness or indifferent eating triggers. Having this knowledge enables us to avoid falling back on bad habits and instead make deliberate decisions.

2. Increased Satisfaction: Mindful eating allows us to appreciate the tastes and richness of our food, which makes smaller servings more satisfying. This can help you lose weight by preventing gluttony.

3. Improved Digestion: By enabling our bodies to assimilate food correctly, eating gradually and thoughtfully improves digestion and lessens symptoms like overfilling and stomach cramps.

4. Emotional Harmony: Eating mindfully helps us distinguish between emotional and physical need for food. When emotional needs are met without the use of food, we create more beneficial coping mechanisms.

5. Enhanced Gratitude: We can develop gratitude and a stronger bond with our food by being mindful of the food we consume, where it emanates from, and the work that goes into preparing it.

Five Techniques for Mindful Eating

1. Begin by being aware: Start by observing your eating patterns without passing judgment. Observe your eating habits—when, where, and why. Is eating something you're doing out of habit, restlessness, or anxiety, or are you really starved?

2. Involve Your Senses: Use every sense available to you when you relax to eat. Take note of your food's flavors, feelings, and colors. Give yourself some time to acknowledge the work that went into making your food.

3. Eat Gradually: Take your time and properly chew every bite. In between mouthfuls, set down your dishes and inhale deeply. This lets you savor your food more thoroughly and reduces the speed at which you're eating.

4. Pay Attention to Your Body: Pay attention to your body's indications of starvation and satiation. Eat without feeling too full, but just enough to be satiated. Appreciate the distinction between emotional eating and when you are actually starved.

5. Practice Gratitude: Give thanks for the sustenance your food provides, both prior to eating and at the end of eating. This might be as simple as taking some time to consider how your food gets from the farm to the dining or expressing a sincere appreciation for enjoying a meal.

Four Strategies for Getting Over Obstacles to Mindful Eating

Gaining the ability to eat mindfully requires time and repetition. During the process, obstacles like emotional prompts, disruptions, or the resurgence of old behaviors are common. The following are some methods to get beyond these obstacles:

1. Mindful Pause: Take a moment to practice mindfulness if you're feeling inclined to eat out of restlessness or tension. Consider whether you really need food or whether there is another need that you can attend to in its place.

2. Environment Control: Reduce interruptions during meals to foster a mindful eating atmosphere. If you are dining with others, shut off your devices, sit at an assigned table, and concentrate on the food and conversation.

3. Self-Compassion: Treat yourself with kindness as you go through the adoption of mindful eating habits. If you experience disappointment or find it difficult to eat thoughtfully, accept it without passing judgment and make a fresh commitment to your routine.

4. Practice Often: Mindful eating habits are developed via perseverance. Include mindful eating in your regular routine; begin with one meal per day and work your way up to more.

Ultimately, beyond forty years of age, mindful eating can be a very effective assistance in your quest to lose weight. Adopting this technique can help you develop a healthy connection with food in addition to providing your body with better nourishment. It's important for you to acknowledge the fact that progress, not perfection, is the aim of adopting the habit of mindful eating. Appreciate each attentive bite as a way forward toward your overall well-being.

CHAPTER TWO

The Secret of Strength Training

Any weight loss program must include strength exercise, but it's especially important for people over forty years of age. Our bodies habitually suffer the loss of bone density and muscle mass as we grow older, which lowers our metabolism and impairs our general physical capacity. Strength exercise, on the other hand, can counteract these impacts and have a major positive impact on both your general health and weight reduction process.

Strength training, which is commonly referred to as resistance training is a form of exercise that utilizes resistance bands, body weights, and heavy weighing metals to develop and solidify muscles. By raising your metabolism, building muscle, and enhancing your entire body structure, strength training provides enduring advantages compared to cardiovascular training or aerobic workouts, which are primarily focused on shedding excess body fat.

Four Principal Advantages of Strength Training

1. Increases Metabolism: Increasing your metabolism is among the main advantages of strength exercise. Strength training raises the amount of fat that your body could shed in the process of going after your normal living activities unlike cardiovascular training or aerobic workouts that shed excess body fat only when you're performing the action. The greater your muscle, the higher the amount of calories your body can burn during the day because muscular tissue needs more energy to sustain than fat tissue.

2. Preserve Lean Muscle Mass: As we grow older, we habitually suffer the loss of muscle mass. This might result in an elevated body fat percentage and a reduced metabolism. Strength training stimulates the development and maintenance of muscle, which helps to reverse the process of losing muscle mass as we grow older. You may preserve or even grow your muscle mass by consistently pushing your muscles with resistance training. Achieving the positive result of losing weight, as well as general strength depends on having a muscular mass.

3. Enhances Bone Density: Strength training also has a good effect on bone density, which is particularly advantageous for women over the age of forty. Women are more likely to develop osteoporosis, a disorder marked by fragile and breakable bones, as their estrogen levels drop throughout menopause. By promoting bone development and firmness, strength training, especially weight-bearing exercises like squats, sprints, and weightlifting, can lower the danger of osteoporosis and support bone health.

4. Boosts Working Fitness: Strength training boosts the capacity to carry out daily duties and pursuits effortlessly. This benefit extends above weight loss. Your stability, stretchability, and general movement will all get better as a result of stronger muscles and joints, which also lowers your chance of falls and accidents as you grow older. Enhanced working fitness not only improves your entire well-being but also facilitates participation in various physical activities.

Five Ways to Include Strength Training in Your Daily Routine

A balanced exercise program that incorporates both strength training and cardiovascular training is necessary to fully reap the rewards of strength training. The following advice can help you include strength training in your weight loss regimen:

1. Start Slowly: To avoid the possibility of getting injured, begin strength training with modest weights if you're new to the sport or haven't worked out in a while. Increase the challenge and dimensions slowly as your strength and self-assurance grow.

2. Pay Attention to Compound Exercises: These exercises are great for burning calories and strengthening many muscle groups at once. Squats, weightlifting, push-ups, and rows are a few examples of compound exercises.

3. Use Resistance Bands: These devices are portable and adaptable, and they may give your strength training regimen some variation. They give you resistance and a complete range of motion during the exercise, which will help you gain muscle and increase your stretchability.

4. Incorporate Rest Days: Include some resting days in your exercise regimen to give your muscles a chance to heal and regenerate. For the best possible recuperation and muscular development, try to take a minimum of forty-eight hours off from your last strength training session to another.

5. Seek Professional Advice: If you're inexperienced in strength training or have certain health problems, you might want to contemplate employing the services of a licensed personal trainer. A trainer can design a workout program specifically for you based on your objectives and skill level, guaranteeing efficient and safe advancement.

You may enhance your general health, movement, and standard of life well into your forties and above by including strength training in your weight loss plan and enjoying its many rewards. Strength training can help you lose those extra pounds as well. It's important for you to acknowledge the fact that perseverance and commitment are necessary to get long-lasting effects, so stick to your exercise regimen and get the life-changing advantages of strength training.

CHAPTER THREE

The Secret of Cardiovascular Exercise for Women over Forty Years

Any weight loss plan must include cardiovascular exercise, but it is mostly important for women over the age of forty. Our metabolism decreases as we get older, which makes losing extra weight harder. However adding frequent cardiovascular exercises to your regimen can assist in boosting your metabolism, strengthen your heart, and make a big difference in your general health.

Five Main Reasons Why Cardiovascular Exercise Is Important for Women Over Forty

Any action that raises your heart rate and improves blood flow is referred to as cardiovascular exercise, sometimes known as aerobic or cardio exercise. Consistent aerobic exercise has several advantages for women over the age of forty, such as:

1. Better Heart Health: As we grow older, the danger of heart disease increases, but cardio workouts also help to toughen your heart muscles, reduce blood pressure, and ultimately decrease your chances of getting heart disease.

2. Enhanced Metabolism: Frequent aerobic exercise increases metabolism, which facilitates effective calorie burning and weight management.

3. Improved Mood: Engaging in cardiovascular activity can cause the production of endorphins, a naturally existing morphine-like substance that makes people feel good, and has the power to elevate mood, lower stress levels, and lessen the signs and symptoms of distress and melancholy.

4. Better Sleep: Sleep issues are a common problem for women over the age of forty. Cardiovascular exercise can assist individuals to sleep more soundly and manage sleep cycles.

5. Enhanced Energy: Consistent aerobic exercise can increase your energy levels, strengthen your stamina, and alleviate the difficulty of daily duties.

Six Types of Cardiovascular Workouts for Women Over the Age of Forty

Take into account your interests, current health concerns, and degree of fitness while choosing your aerobic workouts. The following six moderate and productive aerobic exercises are appropriate for women over the age of forty:

1. Brisk Walking: You may engage in an easy and productive cardio workout of walking practically anywhere and at any time. In order to increase the effectiveness of walking as a cardiovascular exercise, it's important to try to get a minimum of thirty minutes of brisk walking nearly all days of the week.

2. Cycling: Notwithstanding whether you do it outside or on an immovable cycle, cycling is an excellent way to raise your heart rate without straining your joints. It's a good cardiovascular exercise for women over the age of forty years.

3. Swimming: This whole-body exercise is easy on the joints and has great cardiovascular effects. It's mostly helpful for people who have arthritis or joint pain.

4. Dancing: Take up a class or just groove at home to your cherished music. Dancing gives your exercise program an enjoyable twist in addition to raising your heart rate. It's a good cardiovascular exercise for women over the age of forty years.

5. Elliptical Training: Utilizing an elliptical machine offers a moderate approach to working different muscle groups and improving cardiovascular fitness.

6. Group Exercise Programs: For an inspiring and sociable workout, think about enrolling in group exercise programs such as cardio kickboxing, Zumba, or aerobics.

Six Ways to Include Cardio Exercises in Your Daily Routine

You should target a minimum of 150 minutes of moderate-intensity cardio workout every week, distributed across many days, to get the most out of cardiovascular activity. The following six pointers will help you include aerobic exercises in your daily routine:

1. Establish Achievable Goals: Grow the period and magnitude of your workouts slowly, starting with achievable goals in accordance with your present fitness level.

2. Mix It Up: In order to maintain an engaging and interesting workout routine, you can spice it up with various kinds of aerobic exercise programs.

3. Plan Regular Sessions: To guarantee persistence, plan your cardio exercises into your weekly agenda and handle them as appointments.

4. Preparation: Always start your cardio workout with a warm-up to get your muscles ready, and finish with a cool-down to aid in your body's recovery.

5. Pay Attention to Your Body: Observe how exercise affects your body. Adjust your exercise regimen or get advice from a fitness expert if you feel pain or misery.

6. Stay Hydrated: To ensure peak performance, stay hydrated by drinking lots of water prior to, during, and following your workouts.

In conclusion, cardiovascular exercise is an essential part of any program designed to help women over the age of forty lose weight. Your heart health, metabolism, ability to control your weight, and general health can all be improved with consistent cardiac exercise and positive lifestyle decisions. Before beginning any new workout regimen, remember to speak with a healthcare provider or fitness specialist, particularly if you have any hidden health issues. Maintain your motivation and perseverance while having fun in the process to a better-looking appearance.

CHAPTER FOUR

The Secret of Commensurate Sleep and Stress Control

Two sometimes disregarded but crucial components in the fight against weight gain after turning forty are getting enough sleep and controlling stress. These components are essential for sustaining general health and energy as well as for losing excess weight. Let's explore their significance and how you might include them in your weight loss program.

Four Reasons Why Getting Enough Sleep Is Essential for Efficient Weight Loss

There's a good reason why getting enough sleep is crucial for good health. Your body heals, regenerates, and restores stabilization to a number of physiological functions while you sleep. For successful weight control, getting enough sleep is essential for the following four reasons:

1. Hormonal Balance: Ghrelin and leptin, two hormones linked to appetite and fullness, are significantly regulated by commensurate sleep. This equilibrium is upset by getting too little sleep, which increases appetite and cravings for harmful meals.

2. Metabolism: Commensurate sleep guarantees effective energy conservation and usage, which promotes a vigorous metabolism. Conversely, lack of sleep can weaken your metabolism and render it more difficult to reduce body weight.

3. Mental Purity: Relaxed minds are better able to regulate portions and make wise dietary selections. Poor meal preparations and reckless eating are frequently caused by sleep deprivation.

4. Stress Minimization: Stress alleviation and sound sleep are closely related. Your body is more disposed to handle everyday pressures when you get enough sleep, which helps to reduce stress-related weight gain.

Four Methods to Get More Restful Sleep

1. Create a Habit: Endeavor to maintain a regular sleeping pattern by going to sleep and getting out of bed at the same times every day.

2. Establish a Calm Environment: Maintain a cold, dark, and silent bedroom to promote restful sleep. Endeavor to get pillows and a mattress that are more adapted to restful sleep.

3. Limit Screen Time: Melatonin are hormone that the brain produces in response to darkness, and it protects people from the problem of delayed sleep-wake phase disorder, a situation where individuals find it difficult to sleep until about 2 am. Unfortunately, when individuals expose themselves to computer, phone, and tablet screens at night, the production of melatonin hormone will be disrupted. It is therefore important for people to avoid exposing themselves to computer, phone, and tablet screens at least one hour before bedtime in order to promote better sleep.

4. Use Relaxation Techniques: Read a book, stretch gently, meditate, or practice deep breathing exercises to unwind before going to bed.

Four Reasons Why Stress Control is Necessary for Losing Weight After the Age of Forty Years

Prolonged stress affects your physical and mental health as well as your weight and emotional state of mind. The following four factors demonstrate why effective stress management is crucial for losing weight after the age of forty:

1. Cortisol and Weight Gain: Stress leads to the release of cortisol hormone, which has been connected to a higher storage of fat in the abdomen. Relentless stress might lead to difficult-to-lose belly fat.

2. Emotional Eating: When faced with stress, a lot of people turn to food for solace, which can result in overindulging and poor food selections.

3. Sleep Quality: Stress can result in sleep disorders, which can lead to a dangerous cycle in which stress is made worse by inadequate sleep and vice versa.

4. Inflammation: Extended periods of stress could result in systemic inflammation that could cause a number of health problems, including metabolic abnormalities and excess weight.

Four Principal Techniques for Controlling Stress

1. Consistent Exercise: In order to achieve the aim of lowering stress and increasing the release of endorphins, which are hormones that improve mood, it's important to partake in any aerobic exercise that you enjoy, such as dancing, yoga, or brisk walking.

2. Mindfulness and Meditation: It's critical to practice mindfulness exercises and meditation in order to cultivate a state of calmness and immunity to the negative effects of stress.

3. Healthy Coping Mechanisms: Seek out constructive ways to release tension, like journaling, conversing with friends, or taking up enjoyable hobbies.

4. Professional Assistance: You should consider seeking professional counseling or treatment for stress in two different circumstances. They include, when stress becomes too much for you to handle and when you need assistance in creating proper coping mechanisms.

Four Ways to Include Stress Reduction and Commensurate Sleep in Your Weight Loss Strategy

Take into consideration the following advice to fully profit from getting enough sleep and controlling your stress in order to lose weight after the age of forty:

1. Make Sleep A Priority: Try to get between seven to nine hours of good sleep every night.

2. Establish a Calm Bedtime Habit: To let your body know it's time to sleep, make a habit of relaxing with peaceful activities prior to going to sleep at night.

3. Put Stress Reduction Techniques into Practice: In order to enhance your general health, include frequent stress alleviation activities in your daily schedule.

4. Track Progress: Maintain a proper record of how sleep and stress levels affect your efforts to lose weight, and make proper adjustments to your strategies accordingly.

When you focus on getting enough sleep and controlling your stress, you will enhance your ability to lose weight as well as improve your general health and standard of living after the age of forty years.

CHAPTER FIVE

The Secret of Modifying Nutrition for Hormone Balance

Our bodies go through lots of alterations as we grow older, particularly with regard to the production and balancing of hormones. Hormones are essential for energy, mood, metabolism, and general health. Modifying nutrition for hormone balance is essential for weight loss in adults over the age of forty who want to see long-lasting outcomes. We'll explore nutritional approaches that can promote hormonal balance and facilitate the process of losing weight in this chapter.

Five Principal Hormones that are Affected by Age

Prior to discussing nutrition choices, it's critical to comprehend the hormonal alterations that come with aging, especially around the age of forty. Among the major hormones impacted are:

1. Insulin: As we grow older, our response to insulin happens to decline, increasing our danger of insulin resistance and accumulation of excess fat, particularly in the abdominal region.

2. Cortisol: Prolonged stress can raise the levels of cortisol hormone in the body, which can lead to the accumulation of fat, especially around the abdomen.

3. Estrogen and Progesterone: At the time of perimenopause and menopause, the levels of estrogen and progesterone hormone in the body of most women fluctuate, which might have an effect on body constituents and metabolism.

4. Testosterone: As people grow older, their levels of testosterone decrease, which may have an impact on their circulation of fat and muscle mass.

5. Thyroid Hormones: Modifications in thyroid function also have the ability to affect energy levels and metabolism.

Let's now investigate how modifying the things we consume could assist in maintaining hormonal balance for the promotion of weight loss.

Three Macronutrients to Balance Hormones

Hormone control and general health depend on well-proportioned macronutrient consumption. Here's how to maximize the amount of macronutrients you eat:

1. Protein: Make sure your meals contain lean protein sources including fish, poultry, tofu, and lentils. Protein enables an individual to feel satisfied with food easily, assisting in maintaining muscular mass. Again, proteins are needed for the production of hormones.

2. Healthy Fats: Healthy fats assist in the production of hormones and the assimilation of fat-soluble vitamins. They can be obtained from nuts, seeds, avocados, fatty fish, and olive oil.

3. Complex Carbohydrates: Desist from the habit of consuming processed carbohydrates and opt instead for complex carbohydrates like those found in whole grains, fruits, vegetables, and legumes. These give you long-lasting energy, fiber, and vital nutrients without shooting up your blood sugar.

Four Methods for Maintaining Blood Sugar Levels for Hormone Balance

Blood sugar stability is essential for insulin synthesis and hormone balance. In order to maximize blood sugar regulation, the following four practices are essential:

1. Eat Frequently: To avoid blood sugar swings, try to have three well-balanced meals and two snacks each day.

2. Select Low-Glycemic Foods: To prevent abrupt elevations in blood sugar levels, select foods with a low glycemic index, such as leafy greens, quinoa, sweet potatoes, and berries.

3. Limit Added Sugars: Because they can alter the response of the body to insulin hormones, reduce your intake of sweetened beverages, meals, and processed foods.

4. Incorporate Fiber: Foods high in fiber, such as fruits, vegetables, whole grains, and legumes, aid in lowering blood sugar, promoting gut health, and slowing down digestion.

Three Key Techniques for Cortisol and Stress Control

Prolonged stress can result in uncontrolled cortisol levels, which can affect general health and weight control. The following are the three main methods for controlling cortisol and stress:

1. Practice Mindfulness: To encourage relaxation and lower stress, try yoga, tai chi, meditation, or deep breathing techniques.

2. Make Sleep a Priority: To promote hormone balance, metabolic rate, and recuperation, aim for between seven to nine hours of good sleep every night.

3. Physical Activity: Include consistent exercise in your daily schedule, concentrating on enjoyable activities like dance, brisk walking, cycling, as well as resistance training. Exercise elevates mood and reduces cortisol levels.

Five Nutrients to Help Maintain Hormonal Balance

Maintaining hormonal balance requires a number of nutrients. Think about consuming the five nutrients listed below in your diet to maintain hormonal balance and gain the ability to lose weight:

1. Omega-3 Fatty Acids: This nutrient boosts the production of hormones and prevents inflammation. They can be obtained from flaxseeds, chia seeds, walnuts, and fatty fish.

2. Vitamin D: A sufficient quantity of vitamin D in the body assists in the production of hormones and optimum metabolic rate. They can be obtained by spending time in the sun and eating foods high in vitamin D, such as egg yolks, dairy products, and fatty fish.

3. Magnesium: This nutrient promotes calmness of the mind and body, helping to control the levels of cortisol hormones in the body. They can be obtained from whole grains, nuts, seeds, and leafy greens.

4. B vitamins: This nutrient assists hormone balance, mood stability, and the synthesis of energy. They can be obtained from legumes, leafy greens, fish, chicken, and eggs.

5. Probiotics: This nutrient assists in maintaining gut health, which is important for proper hormone metabolism. They can be obtained from yogurt, kefir, sauerkraut, and kimchi.

The Effect of Meal Preparation and Portion Control on Hormone Balance and Weight Loss

Lastly, meal preparation and portion management are crucial components of maximizing nutrition for hormone balance and weight reduction. Here are three key points to note in the effect of meal preparation and portion control on hormone balance and weight loss:

1. Plan Balanced Meals: Each meal should consist of a range of nutrient-dense foods, with an emphasis on vegetables, lean protein, healthy fats, and carbohydrates high in fiber.

2. Exercise Portion Control: Pay attention to serving sizes, particularly when consuming foods high in calories, to prevent overindulging.

3. Remain Hydrated: To promote healthy digestion, metabolic rate, and general well-being, sip a sufficient amount of water all through the day.

By putting these hormone-balanced nutrition methods into practice, people over the age of forty can assist their bodies to lose weight while fostering general health and vigor. Never forget to get advice from a qualified dietician or healthcare provider for individualized suggestions based on your unique requirements and state of health.

CHAPTER SIX

The Secret of Proper Hydration

Our bodies alter as we get older, changing things like our metabolic rate and hormone levels. These alterations may affect our capacity to control our weight. Drinking enough water is one weight control strategy that is frequently disregarded, particularly for people over the age of forty. This chapter will discuss the value of being hydrated and how it affects weight control techniques.

The process of keeping the body's water levels sufficient to maintain several operations in the body is referred to as hydration. Almost all of the body's processes, including the breaking down of food, assimilation of nutrients, circulation of blood, control of body temperature, and waste elimination, depend on water. These functions may be hampered by dehydration, which can result in a number of health problems.

Four Ways Hydration Is Important for Controlling Weight

1. Control Your Appetite: Sometimes people confuse thirst with hunger, which causes them to eat extra calories. Maintaining adequate hydration can help control hunger and stop overindulging.

2. Increase in Metabolic Rate: Studies indicate that consuming water may momentarily increase metabolic rate. A body that is properly hydrated burns calories more effectively, which can assist in losing weight.

3. Water Retention: Ironically, the body's attempt to retain fluids in reaction to thirst can result in water retention if you don't drink a sufficient quantity of water. This may cause an individual to put on weight temporarily.

4. Energy Levels: Being dehydrated might make you tired and less physically fit. We are unable to exercise when we are fatigued, which is important for controlling our weight.

Seven Useful Counsels for Staying Hydrated and Controlling Your Weight

1. Drink Plenty of Water: If you live in a hot area or live a physically active life, try to drink a minimum of eight to ten glasses of water every day.

2. Select Foods High in Water: There are certain foods that are high in water content, which you can include in your diet. Some examples of this kind of food include watermelon, oranges, cucumbers, and tomatoes.

3. Keep an Eye on Urine Color: Frequently assess the hue of your pee. While darker pee may suggest dehydration, pale yellow urine shows adequate hydration.

4. Restrict Sugary Drinks: Sugary beverages result in dehydration and weight gain because it causes the cells of the body to absorb more water. So, restrict the intake of sugary beverages such as soda and juices with added sugar.

5. Have a Glass of Water Before Meals: Drinking water prior to meals might make you feel satiated earlier and assist you in avoiding overindulging.

6. Use a Hydration Tracker: In order to keep a record of your daily water intake and be responsible for the habit of drinking sufficient water, think about utilizing a hydration tracker or app.

7. Be Careful of Alcohol and Caffeine: Due to their potential diuretic properties, alcohol, and caffeinated drinks should be used in moderation and in support of the consumption of enough water.

In conclusion, maintaining enough hydration is essential for good health and is particularly important for people over the age of forty who are trying to lose weight. You may assist your body to lose weight and support a healthy lifestyle by drinking enough water and ensuring to remain hydrated all through the day. Keep in mind that even minor adjustments to your hydration routine can have a big impact on your health.

CHAPTER SEVEN

The Secret of Mind-Body Practices

Our bodies evolve during our lives in a variety of ways, particularly when we grow to the age of forty and above. During this stage, many people start to worry a lot about managing their weight. Nevertheless, conventional methods frequently ignore the strong link between the mind and body in favor of concentrating only on nutrition and exercise. We will examine the function of mind-body techniques in long-term weight loss beyond forty years of age in this chapter.

'Mind-body connection' refers to the intricate relationship that exists between our physical, mental, and emotional well-being. Studies have indicated that our emotional condition has a big influence on our actions, like how we eat, how much we exercise, and how we live our lives in general. By making the most of this relationship, we can develop wholesome routines and see long-lasting weight reduction outcomes.

Four Mindfulness Methods to Encourage Long-Term Weight Loss

The practice of mindfulness is focusing attention on the here and now without passing judgment. In terms of eating, mindfulness can assist us in becoming more cognizant of the foods we choose, the way we eat, and the signs of hunger. The following four mindfulness practices can help with long-term weight reduction:

1. Mindful Eating: Give each bite of food your full attention, noticing its tastes, textures, and impressions. Endeavor to steer clear of distractions like using a mobile phone or laptop while eating, and avoid eating while walking or driving.

2. Hunger Awareness: Acquire the ability to distinguish between emotional and real hunger. Ask yourself whether you are genuinely hungry or just looking for a way to console yourself with a meal.

3. Portion Control: In order to prevent overindulging, portion food mindfully by using tiny plates. Pay attention to your body's satiation cues and quit eating when you're contented, and not until you're jam-packed with food.

4. Emotional Control: In order to control your emotions without resorting to eating, use mindfulness-based stress-reduction practices. You can use techniques such as deep breathing, meditation, or mild yoga to buttress your emotional harmony.

Four Methods for Fostering a Positive Body Image

The way we feel about our bodies affects how we feel about food and activity. Unhealthy habits that can not be sustained over a long-term period such as restrictive diet or excessive exercise, might be brought on by a negative body image. The following four techniques can help you develop a good body image:

1. Self-Compassion: Show yourself care and empathy, especially when you experience obstacles or disappointments in your struggle to lose weight.

2. Gratitude Practice: Pay more attention to your body's capabilities than its outward look. Give thanks for your body's toughness, strength, and capacity to assist you with daily tasks.

3. Acceptance: Instead of focusing on reaching a particular weight or size, accept your body for what it is and realize that real health and comfort emanate from self-love and self-care.

4. Body-Positive Environment: Assemble a network of uplifting individuals who celebrate variety and advocate for body positivity. Restrict your exposure to the media and social factors that uphold an unattainable degree of beauty.

Four Methods for Combining Mindfulness and Movement

Losing weight requires exercise, but exercise must not be boring or hard. It is possible to increase the sustainability and enjoyment of physical activity by combining movement and mindfulness. The following four methods integrate mindfulness with movement:

1. Mindful Movement: Take part in exercises that emphasize stretchability, stability, and the mind-body connection, such as yoga, tai chi, or qigong. These exercises can aid with stress reduction, posture correction, and improvement of body awareness.

2. Take Mindful Nature Walks: As you stroll through the outdoors, focus on the sights, sounds, and feelings that surround you. Make a connection with nature to improve your general health.

3. Joyful Exercise: Embrace the kind of exercise that makes you happy and content such as cycling, gardening, brisk walking, swimming, or dancing. Try to find methods to enjoy exercising instead of viewing it as a task.

4. Mindful Rest: Establish a harmony between movement and commensurate rest and relaxation. In order to encourage general relaxation and restoration, try relaxation techniques like gradual muscle relaxation, guided visualization, or mild stretching.

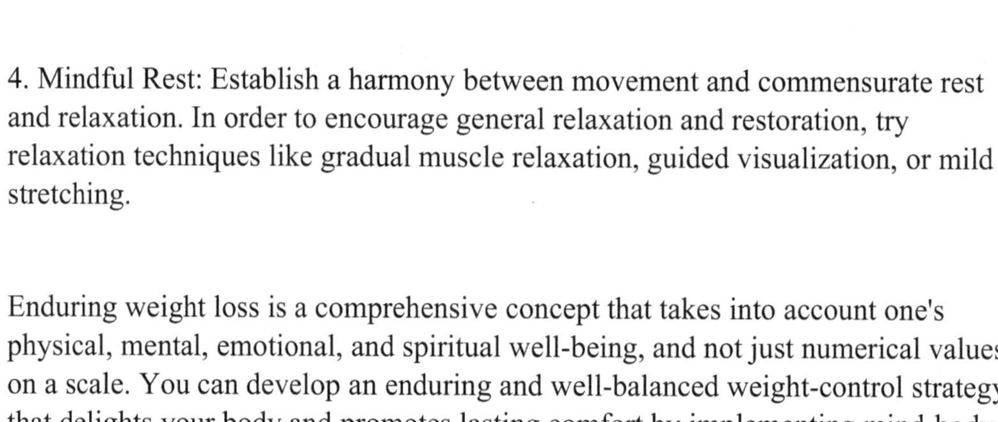

Enduring weight loss is a comprehensive concept that takes into account one's physical, mental, emotional, and spiritual well-being, and not just numerical values on a scale. You can develop an enduring and well-balanced weight-control strategy that delights your body and promotes lasting comfort by implementing mind-body techniques.

In summary, mind-body techniques are essential for attaining long-term weight loss beyond the age of forty. Through the practice of mindfulness, body positivity, movement integration, and holistic well-being, you may design a customized weight-control strategy that will benefit your mind, body, and soul for the rest of your entire life.

CHAPTER EIGHT

The Secret of Beating Periods Of Little Change

You've probably felt both the joy of accomplishment and the annoyance of reaching a weight reduction plateau by this point. It might be discouraging to experience plateaus, which are typical, especially as we grow older. They are not unbeatable, though. We'll look at practical methods in this chapter for beating weight reduction plateaus and keeping up the process of losing weight beyond the age of forty.

There Are Three Causes of Weight Loss Plateaus

Prior to delving into tactics, it's critical to comprehend plateaus and their causes. When you keep trying to lose weight but your weight doesn't move, it's called a weight loss plateau. Three factors frequently lead to plateaus, including:

1. Metabolic Adaptation: When weight loss occurs, your metabolic rate changes, resulting in a decreased resting energy expenditure.

2. Water Retention: Variations in this property may conceal weight loss due to fat.

3. Diminished Caloric Shortfall: As your body adjusts to your latest eating pattern, the initial calorie shortfall may no longer be as productive.

Let's now discuss the five main methods that women over forty might use to break through weight reduction plateaus:

1. Reevaluate Your Calorie Intake: Reevaluating your calorie intake is among the first steps in getting past a plateau. It's possible that your body has adjusted to your existing calorie intake over time, making more weight reduction difficult. In order to overcome the challenge, attempt the following three strategies:

a. Recalculate Your TDEE: TDEE is an acronym, where T stands for Total, D stands for Daily, E stands for Energy, and E stands for Expenditure. In order to discover the value of your TDEE, use an internet calculator assigned for that purpose. Then, modify your calorie intake in accordance with your new TDEE.

b. Monitor Your Food Intake: Take careful note of what you consume to make sure you're not getting in greater calories than you assume.

c. Take a Look at the Calorie Cycling Approach: In order to avoid metabolic adaptation, oscillate between days with greater and lower calorie consumption.

2. Adjust Your Workout Pattern: If you have been exercising in a certain pattern for a long time, your body might have gotten used to it and you've reached a plateau. To overcome the challenge, attempt the following three strategies:

a. Try High-Intensity Interval Training (HIIT): Include HIIT exercises to increase your metabolic rate and burn more calories.

b. Strength Training: Grow your muscle mass with strength training exercises to overcome plateaus and raise your resting metabolic rate.

c. Add Variety: In order to keep your exercising activities ambitious and interesting, mix up your routines by adding new exercises, classes, or outdoor activities.

3. Make Stress Management and Sleep a Priority: Stress reduction and commensurate sleep are important factors in the pursuit of the goal of losing weight. Focus on the following three areas to improve your overall health and get past sleep deprivation and stress management-related plateaus:

a. Make Quality Sleep a Priority: In order to maximize hormone balance and restoration, endeavor to get between seven to nine hours of good sleep every night.

b. Use Stress Reduction Techniques: In order to control stress successfully, include stress reduction techniques such as mindfulness, meditation, yoga, or deep breathing exercises in your daily routine.

c. Make Sure to Take Days Off: In order to avoid fatigue, give your body enough time to relax and heal from physical activities.

4. Examine Your Macronutrient Balance: Modifying your macronutrient proportions can occasionally spur weight loss. Take into consideration these three modifications to get beyond plateaus caused by the balance of macronutrients:

a. Boost Protein Intake: Protein assists in losing weight by promoting satiety and maintaining lean muscle mass.

b. Adjust Your Intake of Carbohydrates and Fats: Try out various carbohydrate and fat ratios to see what your body responds to the best.

c. Embrace Nutrient-Dense Foods: To promote general health and weight control, select whole foods high in nutrients.

5. Remain Consistent and Patient: Lastly, keep in mind that perseverance and consistency are necessary to break through plateaus. Steer clear of excessive diets or aggressive measures that offer fast cures. Instead, concentrate on enduring, pragmatic practices that you can stick to. Learn to appreciate accomplishments that are not related to your weighing numbers including more vitality, better fit in clothes, and general health.

In summary, it's important for you to understand that plateaus are a normal part of the process of losing weight, especially as we become older. After the age of forty, you can continue to lose weight by beating plateaus by making smart changes to your diet, exercise regimen, sleep schedule, and stress management techniques. Mastering the variables that contribute to plateaus will help you achieve your goals. It's important for you to remain devoted, and consistent, and have faith in the process of losing weight.

CHAPTER NINE

The Secret of Developing a Supportive Environment

Beyond the age of forty, losing weight can be a difficult process, but you must not do it without the assistance of others. Essentially, you may greatly improve your probability of success by establishing a supportive environment and encompassing yourself with like-minded people. We'll discuss the value of creating a network that supports you in your weight reduction efforts in this chapter, along with strategies for doing so.

Four Strategies for Creating a Helpful Environment

Your surroundings have a significant impact on the habits, behaviors, and, eventually, weight loss success that you achieve. Establishing a supportive environment entails positioning oneself for success by lowering barriers to healthy living and increasing accessibility to healthy decisions.

1. Arrange Your Living Area: To begin, arrange your living area in a way that encourages a healthy lifestyle. Fill up your kitchen with wholesome items like whole grains, lean meats, and fresh produce for maximum nutrition. Get rid of any bad snacks or temptations that could prevent you from making progress in your weight loss endeavor.

2. Establish a Home Gym or Exercise Area: Ideally, reserve a room in your house for physical activity. This might be a tiny home workout center furnished with simple tools like yoga mats, resistance bands, and weights. Maintaining

consistency in your exercise program is much easier when you have a convenient area to exercise.

3. Establish a Meal Prep System: The idea of establishing a meal prep system is to make the planning of your meal easy without much mental activity. Every week, set aside some time to plan and prepare wholesome meals and appetizers. In order to make it simple to access wholesome selections on hectic days, spend money on high-quality food storage containers.

4. Decrease Stress and Enhance Sleep: Creating a supportive atmosphere also entails stress management and putting a high priority on restful sleep. Establish a calming evening routine, restrict screen time prior to going to sleep, and engage in stress-relieving techniques such as deep breathing and mindfulness.

Four Strategies for Growing a Helpful Community

In the entire process of your weight loss endeavor, encompassing oneself with a supportive group can offer inducement, responsibility, and exhortation on the farther side of your physical surroundings.

1. Establish Connections with Like-Minded People: Look for people who have similar fitness and health-related objectives and ideals. Participate in local gathering groups, social media platforms, or online forums devoted to exercise, healthy living, or weight loss. These groups can provide priceless companionship, support, and guidance.

2. Involve Your Friends and Family: Ask your close friends and family for support by sharing your goals with them. Ask children to participate with you in health-promoting activities like cooking healthy meals, taking walks working out, or

examining new exercise regimens. Having supportive family and friends can make a big impact on your weight loss endeavor.

3. Collaborate with a Supportive Healthcare Team: Take into account collaborating with a healthcare team that is aware of your unique requirements and obstacles. A certified nutritionist, personal trainer, psychiatrist, or other experts who may offer direction, support, and responsibility may fall under this category.

4. Honor Every Little Progress: Congratulate yourself on any accomplishment, irrespective of the size, and let your group of supporters know about it. Achieving a goal in weight reduction, increasing your level of fitness, or forming healthy habits all require acknowledgment of your achievement, which inspires and builds confidence.

Though creating a community and supportive atmosphere can be quite helpful, it's important to recognize that obstacles can appear along the path. Remain strong and rely on your network of support when things get tough. It's important for you to acknowledge the fact that obstacles are a normal part of any worthwhile goal, and the thing that counts the most is that you overcome them and get going.

You will be more equipped to handle the vicissitudes of weight loss after the age of forty with confidence and tenacity if you develop a supportive environment and encompass yourself with positive people. As you strive toward a healthier, happier version of yourself, adopt the power of teamwork, support, and common objectives.

CHAPTER TEN

The Secret of Perseverance

You've probably noticed by now that crash diets and quick cures are not the best approach to losing weight in a lasting way. It's about accepting patience and consistency as the cornerstones of your new lifestyle. We'll go into more detail in this chapter on the importance of patience and consistency as well as how to develop these traits in order to successfully lose weight.

Four Reasons Why Maintaining Consistency Is Crucial to Weight Loss

The secret to enduring success in any activity, including weight loss, is consistency. It all comes down to creating tiny, long-lasting habits that you follow every day. Here are four explanations of why maintaining a consistent weight loss plan is important:

1. Develop behaviors: Being consistent aids in the formation of new behaviors that will aid in your weight loss efforts. Consistently exercising, eating well-balanced meals, and engaging in mindful eating are all examples of behaviors that become automatic through repetition.

2. Stabilizes Motivation: Although motivation varies, perseverance helps you stay motivated even when it starts to wane. You can develop an awareness of discipline that gets you through difficult times by making an effort to follow a routine.

3. Produces Predictable Outcomes: Reliable activities have predictable outcomes. You'll see moderate but constant progress toward your objectives of losing weight when you consistently adhere to a healthy diet and exercise regimen.

4. Enhances Responsibility: Maintaining consistency increases your self-responsibility. Adhering to a plan and maintaining it shows that you are responsible for your decisions and results, which promotes a productive attitude.

Four Techniques to Adopt Consistency for Losing Weight

1. Establish Realistic Goals: Divide your objectives for weight loss into achievable benchmarks. Instead of targetting overnight huge changes, concentrate on gradual progress on a regular basis.

2. Establish a Routine: Make a daily or weekly plan that allows time for self-care, workout, and meal preparation. Maintaining a schedule facilitates staying on course.

3. Monitor Your Progress: Record your food consumption, workouts, and advancement in your weight loss goal. Keep track of changes and make any adjustments to your strategy using a spreadsheet, journal, or app.

4. Remain Adaptable: Although consistency is crucial, it's also critical to remain adaptable and adjust to obstacles or disappointments. If things fail to go according to plan, try not to blame yourself much and instead concentrate on moving in the right direction.

Four Reasons Why Patience is Important for Losing Weight

Another essential component of effective weight loss, particularly as we grow older, is patience. It's about realizing that growth might not always be straightforward and that enduring changes require time. The following four factors highlight the importance of patience when attempting to lose weight:

1. Allows for Reliable Changes: Recovered weight gain or unmanageable behaviors are frequently the result of rapid weight loss. You may create enduring habits by making small, reliable adjustments with patience.

2. Lessens Stress: Stress can undermine your attempts to lose weight. Impatience and irrational expectations can cause stress. Even when you hit a wall or have a slow period of growth, patience keeps you composed and focused.

3. Enhances Mental Health: Learning to be patient fosters self-compassion and a good outlook. Rather than becoming disheartened or condemning, you learn to find joy in little accomplishments and maintain your motivation over time.

4. Promotes Learning and Adaptation: Having patience allows you to reflect on your past experiences and modify your strategy. It's a voyage of mental and physical contemplation and development.

Four Methods for Developing Patience in Order to Lose Weight

1. Establish Reasonable Timetables: Recognize that long-term, sustained weight loss takes time. Stay away from impractical timelines and quick turnaround times as these can irritate people.

2. Put an Emphasis on Non-Scale Victories: Honor accomplishments that go beyond the numbers on a weighing scale such as more vitality, a happier

disposition, better sleep, or more comfortably fitting clothes. These triumphs hold equal significance to the figures on the scale.

3. Engage in Mindfulness Practice: All through your endeavor to lose weight, remain aware and in the now. Pay attention to your body's signals, savor your meals without interruptions, and acknowledge your feelings about food and physical activity.

4. Seek Support: Regardless of whether it's from friends, family, a weight-loss organization, or a professional coach, safeguard yourself with people who are supportive of you. The trip might be less intimidating and more pleasurable when you have friends who support you and appreciate your struggles.

Being patient and being consistent is essential when trying to lose weight. These are enduring traits that enhance your general comfort rather than merely short-term tactics. Accept the process, have faith in your skills, and continue to be dedicated to changing things for the better every day.

Never forget that every step, irrespective of the size, is a stride toward development. Acknowledge your successes, take lessons from failures, and keep going forward with tenacity and fortitude. Every second of consistency and patience you put into being a better, happier version of yourself is worthwhile.

CONCLUSION

For ladies looking for hormone balance and reliable weight loss, this book offers a life-changing adventure. With the help of this little manual, readers have learned important tactics that are grounded in logic and science. Each cardinal secret reveals a roadmap to enduring success, from comprehending hormonal changes to adopting mindful eating practices and a holistic approach to fitness.

We've covered the connections between stress reduction, exercise, sleep, and diet in this book as they relate to reaching ideal health and controlling weight. Women may face the obligations of aging with dignity and energy if they prioritize self-care and put tailored techniques into practice.

Keep in mind that every step you take toward lasting weight loss is a victory as you set out on the process. Accept the journey, acknowledge your accomplishments, and draw lessons from failures. You will lead a longer, healthier, and more satisfying life after the age of forty and beyond if you persevere, commit, and devote yourself to lifetime fitness.